MW01233982

The Complete Mediterranean Dishes Cookbook

*Super Tasty and Quick Recipes
To Improve Your Health*

Alison Russell

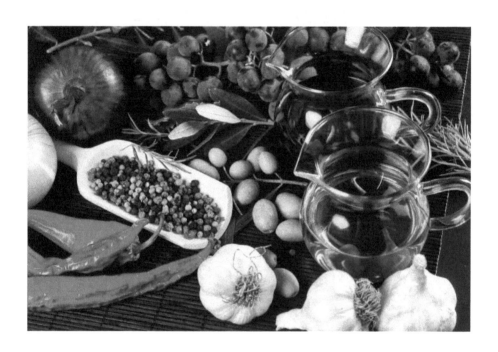

advice. The content within this book has been derived from various sources. Please consult a licensed professional before attempting any techniques outlined in this book.

By reading this document, the reader agrees that under no circumstances is the author responsible for any losses, direct or indirect, which are incurred as a result of the use of information contained within this document, including, but not limited to, — errors, omissions, or inaccuracies.

Table of contents

Breakfast

Spinach and Egg Breakfast Wraps

Prep time: 10 minutes | Cook time: 7 minutes | Serves 2

1 tablespoon olive oil

¼ cup minced onion

3 to 4 tablespoons minced sun-dried tomatoes in olive oil and herbs

3 large eggs, whisked

1½ cups packed baby spinach

1 ounce (28 g) crumbled feta cheese

Salt, to taste

2 (8-inch) whole-wheat tortillas

1. Heat the olive oil in a large skillet over medium-high heat.
2. Sauté the onion and tomatoes for about 3 minutes, stirring occasionally, until softened.
3. Reduce the heat to medium. Add the whisked eggs and stir-fry for 1 to 2 minutes.

4. Stir in the baby spinach and scatter with the crumbled feta cheese. Season as needed with salt.

5. Remove the egg mixture from the heat to a plate. Set aside.

6. Working in batches, place 2 tortillas on a microwave-safe dish and microwave for about 20 seconds to make them warm.

7. Spoon half of the egg mixture into each tortilla. Fold them in half and roll up, then serve.

Per Serving

calories: 434 | fat: 28.1g | protein: 17.2g | carbs: 30.8g | fiber: 6.0g | sodium: 551mg

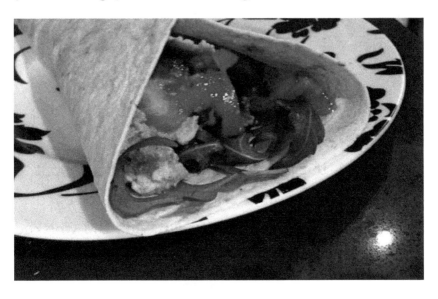

Pumpkin Pie Parfait

Prep time: 5 minutes | Cook time: 0 minutes | Serves 4

1 (15-ounce / 425-g) can pure pumpkin purée

4 teaspoons honey

1 teaspoon pumpkin pie spice

¼ teaspoon ground cinnamon

2 cups plain Greek yogurt

1 cup honey granola

1. Combine the pumpkin purée, honey, pumpkin pie spice, and cinnamon in a large bowl and stir to mix well.
2. Cover the bowl with plastic wrap and chill in the refrigerator for at least 2 hours.
3. Make the parfaits: Layer each parfait glass with ¼ cup pumpkin mixture in the bottom. Top with ¼ cup of yogurt and scatter each top with ¼ cup of honey granola. Repeat the layers until the glasses are full.
4. Serve immediately.

Per Serving

calories: 263 | fat: 8.9g | protein: 15.3g | carbs: 34.6g | fiber: 6.0g | sodium: 91mg

Mediterranean Eggs (Shakshuka)

Prep time: 5 minutes | Cook time: 20 minutes | Serves 4

2 tablespoons extra-virgin olive oil

1 cup chopped shallots

1 teaspoon garlic powder

1 cup finely diced potato

1 cup chopped red bell peppers

1 (14.5-ounce/ 411-g) can diced tomatoes, drained

¼ teaspoon ground cardamom

¼ teaspoon paprika

¼ teaspoon turmeric

4 large eggs

¼ cup chopped fresh cilantro

1. Preheat the oven to 350ºF (180ºC).
2. Heat the olive oil in an ovenproof skillet over medium-high heat until it shimmers.
3. Add the shallots and sauté for about 3 minutes, stirring occasionally, until fragrant.
4. Fold in the garlic powder, potato, and bell peppers and stir to combine.
5. Cover and cook for 10 minutes, stirring frequently.

6. Add the tomatoes, cardamon, paprika, and turmeric and mix well.
7. When the mixture begins to bubble, remove from the heat and crack the eggs into the skillet.
8. Transfer the skillet to the preheated oven and bake for 5 to 10 minutes, or until the egg whites are set and the yolks are cooked to your liking.
9. Remove from the oven and garnish with the cilantro before serving.

Per Serving

calories: 223 | fat: 11.8g | protein: 9.1g | carbs: 19.5g | fiber: 3.0g | sodium: 277mg

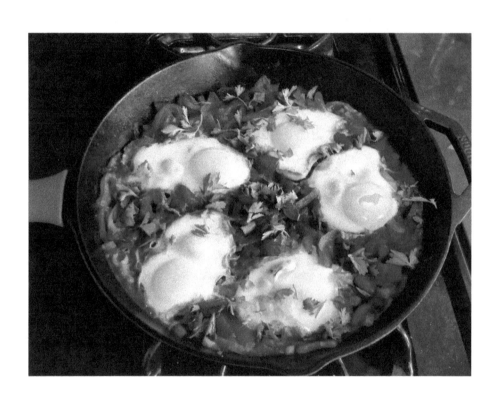

Ricotta Toast with Strawberries

Prep time: 10 minutes | Cook time: 0 minutes | Serves 2

½ cup crumbled ricotta cheese

1 tablespoon honey, plus additional as needed

Pinch of sea salt, plus additional as needed

4 slices of whole-grain bread, toasted

1 cup sliced fresh strawberries

4 large fresh basil leaves, sliced into thin shreds

1. Mix together the cheese, honey, and salt in a small bowl until well incorporated.
2. Taste and add additional salt and honey as needed.
3. Spoon 2 tablespoons of the cheese mixture onto each slice of bread and spread it all over.
4. Sprinkle the sliced strawberry and basil leaves on top before serving.

Per Serving

calories: 274 | fat: 7.9g | protein: 15.1g | carbs: 39.8g | fiber: 5.0g | sodium: 322mg

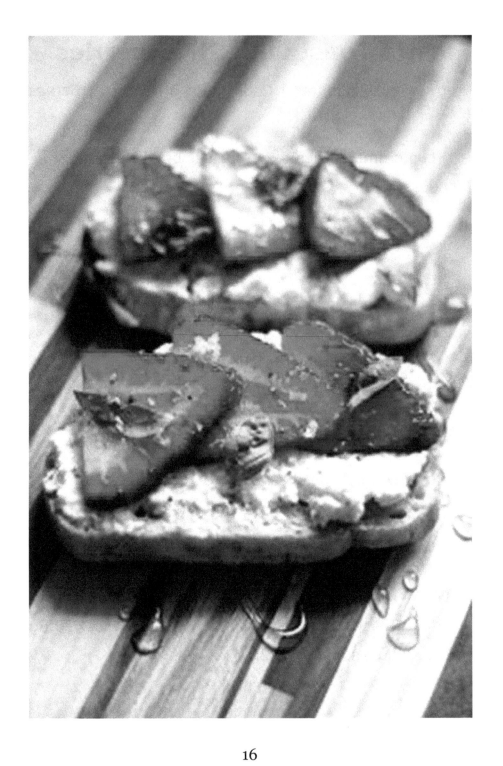

Egg Bake

Prep time: 10 minutes | Cook time: 30 minutes | Serves 2

1 tablespoon olive oil

1 slice whole-grain bread

4 large eggs

3 tablespoons unsweetened almond milk

½ teaspoon onion powder

¼ teaspoon garlic powder

¾ cup chopped cherry tomatoes

¼ teaspoon salt

Pinch freshly ground black pepper

1. Preheat the oven to 375ºF (190ºC).
2. Coat two ramekins with the olive oil and transfer to a baking sheet. Line the bottom of each ramekin with ½ of bread slice.
3. In a medium bowl, whisk together the eggs, almond milk, onion powder, garlic powder, tomatoes, salt, and pepper until well combined.
4. Pour the mixture evenly into two ramekins. Bake in the preheated oven for 30 minutes, or until the eggs are completely set.
5. Cool for 5 minutes before serving.

Per Serving

calories: 240 | fat: 17.4g | protein: 9.0g | carbs: 12.2g | fiber: 2.8g | sodium: 396mg

Creamy Peach Smoothie

Prep time: 15 minutes | Cook time: 0 minutes | Serves 2

2 cups packed frozen peaches, partially thawed

½ ripe avocado

½ cup plain or vanilla Greek yogurt

2 tablespoons flax meal

1 tablespoon honey

1 teaspoon orange extract

1 teaspoon vanilla extract

1. Place all the ingredients in a blender and blend until completely mixed and smooth.
2. Divide the mixture into two bowls and serve immediately.

Per Serving

calories: 212 | fat: 13.1g | protein: 6.0g | carbs: 22.5g | fiber: 7.2g | sodium: 40mg

Blueberry Smoothie

Prep time: 5 minutes | Cook time: 0 minutes | Serves 1

1 cup unsweetened almond milk, plus additional as needed

¼ cup frozen blueberries

2 tablespoons unsweetened almond butter

1 tablespoon extra-virgin olive oil

1 tablespoon ground flaxseed or chia seeds

1 to 2 teaspoons maple syrup

½ teaspoon vanilla extract

¼ teaspoon ground cinnamon

1. Blend all the ingredients in a blender until smooth and creamy.
2. You can add additional almond milk to reach your preferred consistency as needed. Serve immediately.

Per Serving

calories: 459 | fat: 40.1g | protein: 8.9g | carbs: 20.0g | fiber: 10.1g | sodium: 147mg

Cauliflower Breakfast Porridge

Prep time: 5 minutes | Cook time: 5 minutes | Serves 2

2 cups riced cauliflower

¾ cup unsweetened almond milk

4 tablespoons extra-virgin olive oil, divided

2 teaspoons grated fresh orange peel (from ½ orange)

½ teaspoon almond extract or vanilla extract

½ teaspoon ground cinnamon

⅛ teaspoon salt

4 tablespoons chopped walnuts, divided

1 to 2 teaspoons maple syrup (optional)

1. Place the riced cauliflower, almond milk, 2 tablespoons of olive oil, orange peel, almond extract, cinnamon, and salt in a medium saucepan.

2. Stir to incorporate and bring the mixture to a boil over medium-high heat, stirring often.

3. Remove from the heat and add 2 tablespoons of chopped walnuts and maple syrup (if desired).

4. Stir again and divide the porridge into bowls. To serve, sprinkle each bowl evenly with

remaining 2 tablespoons of walnuts and olive oil.

Per Serving

calories: 381 | fat: 37.8g | protein: 5.2g | carbs: 10.9g | fiber: 4.0g | sodium: 228mg

Morning Overnight Oats with Raspberries

Prep time: 5 minutes | Cook time: 0 minutes | Serves 2

²⁄₃ cup unsweetened almond milk

¼ cup raspberries

1⅓ cup rolled oats

1 teaspoon honey

¼ teaspoon turmeric

⅛ teaspoon ground cinnamon

Pinch ground cloves

1. Place the almond milk, raspberries, rolled oats, honey, turmeric, cinnamon, and cloves in a mason jar. Cover and shake to combine.
2. Transfer to the refrigerator for at least 8 hours, preferably 24 hours.
3. Serve chilled.

Per Serving

calories: 81 | fat: 1.9g | protein: 2.1g | carbs: 13.8g | fiber: 3.0g | sodium: 97mg

Tomato and Egg Scramble

Prep time: 10 minutes | Cook time: 20 minutes | Serves 4

2 tablespoons extra-virgin olive oil

¼ cup finely minced red onion

1½ cups chopped fresh tomatoes

2 garlic cloves, minced

½ teaspoon dried thyme

½ teaspoon dried oregano

8 large eggs

½ teaspoon salt

¼ teaspoon freshly ground black pepper

¾ cup crumbled feta cheese

¼ cup chopped fresh mint leaves

1. Heat the olive oil in a large skillet over medium heat.
2. Sauté the red onion and tomatoes in the hot skillet for 10 to 12 minutes, or until the tomatoes are softened.
3. Stir in the garlic, thyme, and oregano and sauté for 2 to 4 minutes, or until the garlic is fragrant.
4. Meanwhile, beat the eggs with the salt and pepper in a medium bowl until frothy.

5. Pour the beaten eggs into the skillet and reduce the heat to low. Scramble for 3 to 4 minutes, stirring constantly, or until the eggs are set.

6. Remove from the heat and scatter with the feta cheese and mint. Serve warm.

Per Serving

calories: 260 | fat: 21.9g | protein: 10.2g | carbs: 5.8g | fiber: 1.0g | sodium: 571mg

Sides, Salads, and Soups

Sumptuous Greek Vegetable Salad

Prep time: 20 minutes | Cook time: 0 minutes | Serves 6

Salad:

1 (15-ounce / 425-g) can chickpeas, drained and rinsed

1 (14-ounce / 397-g) can artichoke hearts, drained and halved

1 head Bibb lettuce, chopped (about 2½ cups)

1 cucumber, peeled deseeded, and chopped (about 1½ cups)

1½ cups grape tomatoes, halved

½ cup cubed feta cheese

Dressing:

1 tablespoon freshly squeezed lemon juice (from about ½ small lemon)

¼ teaspoon freshly ground black pepper

1 tablespoon chopped fresh oregano

2 tablespoons extra-virgin olive oil

1 tablespoon red wine vinegar

1 teaspoon honey

¼ cup chopped basil
leaves

½ cup sliced black
olives

1. Combine the ingredients for the salad in a large salad bowl, then toss to combine well.
2. Combine the ingredients for the dressing in a small bowl, then stir to mix well.
3. Dress the salad and serve immediately.

Per Serving

calories: 165 | fat: 8.1g | protein: 7.2g | carbs: 17.9g | fiber: 7.0g | sodium: 337mg

Brussels Sprout and Apple Slaw

Prep time: 15 minutes | Cook time: 0 minutes | Serves 4

Salad:

1 pound (454 g) Brussels sprouts, stem ends removed and sliced thinly

1 apple, cored and sliced thinly

½ red onion, sliced thinly

Dressing:

1 teaspoon Dijon mustard

2 teaspoons apple cider vinegar

1 tablespoon raw honey

1 cup plain coconut yogurt

1 teaspoon sea salt

For Garnish:

½ cup pomegranate seeds

½ cup chopped toasted hazelnuts

1. Combine the ingredients for the salad in a large salad bowl, then toss to combine well.
2. Combine the ingredients for the dressing in a small bowl, then stir to mix well.
3. Dress the salad let sit for 10 minutes. Serve with pomegranate seeds and toasted hazelnuts on top.

Per Serving

calories: 248 | fat: 11.2g | protein: 12.7g | carbs: 29.9g | fiber: 8.0g | sodium: 645mg

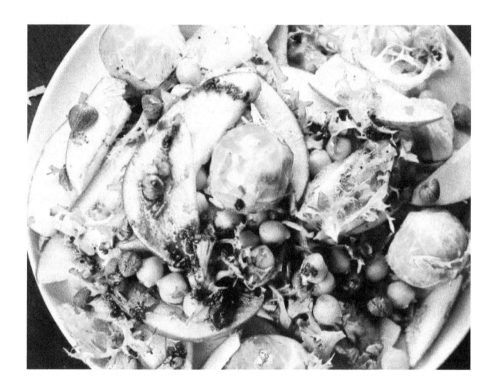

Butternut Squash and Cauliflower Soup

Prep time: 15 minutes | Cook time: 4 hours | Serves 4 to 6

1 pound (454 g) butternut squash, peeled and cut into 1-inch cubes

1 small head cauliflower, cut into 1-inch pieces

1 onion, sliced

2 cups unsweetened coconut milk

1 tablespoon curry powder

½ cup no-added-sugar apple juice

4 cups low-sodium vegetable soup

2 tablespoons coconut oil

1 teaspoon sea salt

¼ teaspoon freshly ground white pepper

¼ cup chopped fresh cilantro, divided

1. Combine all the ingredients, except for the cilantro, in the slow cooker. Stir to mix well.
2. Cook on high heat for 4 hours or until the vegetables are tender.
3. Pour the soup in a food processor, then pulse until creamy and smooth.
4. Pour the puréed soup in a large serving bowl and garnish with cilantro before serving.

Per Serving

calories: 415 | fat: 30.8g | protein: 10.1g | carbs: 29.9g
| fiber: 7.0g | sodium: 1386mg

Cherry, Plum, Artichoke, and Cheese Board

Prep time: 15 minutes | Cook time: 0 minutes | Serves 4

2 cups rinsed cherries

2 cups rinsed and sliced plums

2 cups rinsed carrots, cut into sticks

1 cup canned low-sodium artichoke hearts, rinsed and drained

1 cup cubed feta cheese

1. Arrange all the ingredients in separated portions on a clean board or a large tray, then serve with spoons, knife, and forks.

Per Serving

calories: 417 | fat: 13.8g | protein: 20.1g | carbs: 56.2g | fiber: 3.0g | sodium: 715mg

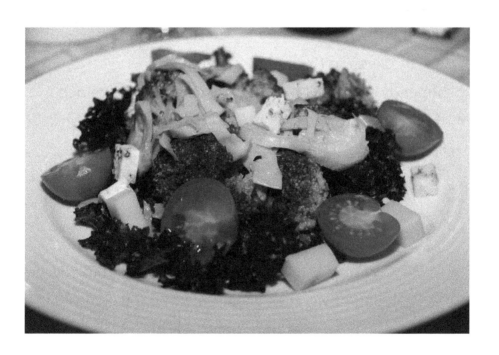

Artichoke and Arugula Salad

Prep time: 10 minutes | Cook time: 0 minutes | Serves 6

Salad:

6 canned oil-packed artichoke hearts, sliced

6 cups baby arugula leaves

6 fresh olives, pitted and chopped

1 cup cherry tomatoes, sliced in half

Dressing:

1 teaspoon Dijon mustard

2 tablespoons balsamic vinegar

1 clove garlic, minced

2 tablespoons extra-virgin olive oil

For Garnish:

4 fresh basil leaves, thinly sliced

1. Combine the ingredients for the salad in a large salad bowl, then toss to combine well.
2. Combine the ingredients for the dressing in a small bowl, then stir to mix well.
3. Dress the salad, then serve with basil leaves on top.

Per Serving

calories: 134 | fat: 12.1g | protein: 1.6g | carbs: 6.2g | fiber: 3.0g| sodium: 65mg

Baby Potato and Olive Salad

Prep time: 10 minutes | Cook time: 20 minutes | Serves 6

2 pounds (907 g) baby potatoes, cut into 1-inch cubes

1 tablespoon low-sodium olive brine

3 tablespoons freshly squeezed lemon juice (from about 1 medium lemon)

¼ teaspoon kosher salt

3 tablespoons extra-virgin olive oil

½ cup sliced olives

2 tablespoons torn fresh mint

1 cup sliced celery (about 2 stalks)

2 tablespoons chopped fresh oregano

1. Put the tomatoes in a saucepan, then pour in enough water to submerge the tomatoes about 1 inch.
2. Bring to a boil over high heat, then reduce the heat to medium-low. Simmer for 14 minutes or until the potatoes are soft.

3. Meanwhile, combine the olive brine, lemon juice, salt, and olive oil in a small bow. Stir to mix well.

4. Transfer the cooked tomatoes in a colander, then rinse with running cold water. Pat dry with paper towels.

5. Transfer the tomatoes in a large salad bowl, then drizzle with olive brine mixture. Spread with remaining ingredients and toss to combine well.

6. Serve immediately.

Per Serving

calories: 220 | fat: 6.1g | protein: 4.3g | carbs: 39.2g | fiber: 5.0g | sodium: 231mg

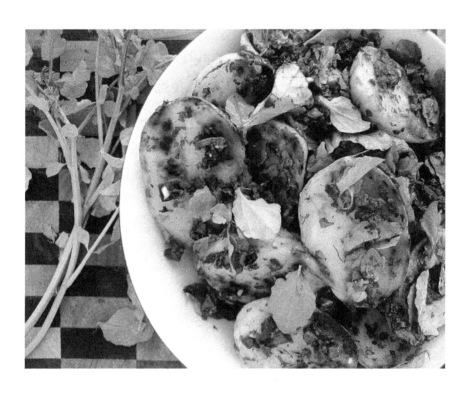

Barley, Parsley, and Pea Salad

Prep time: 10 minutes | Cook time: 10 minutes | Serves 4

2 cups water

1 cup quick-cooking barley

1 small bunch flat-leaf parsley, chopped (about 1 to 1½ cups)

2 cups sugar snap pea pods

Juice of 1 lemon

½ small red onion, diced

2 tablespoons extra-virgin olive oil

Sea salt and freshly ground pepper, to taste

1. Pour the water in a saucepan. Bring to a boil. Add the barley to the saucepan, then put the lid on.
2. Reduce the heat to low. Simmer the barley for 10 minutes or until the liquid is absorbed, then let sit for 5 minutes.
3. Open the lid, then transfer the barley in a colander and rinse under cold running water.
4. Pour the barley in a large salad bowl and add the remaining ingredients. Toss to combine well.
5. Serve immediately.

Per Serving

calories: 152 | fat: 7.4g | protein: 3.7g | carbs: 19.3g | fiber: 4.7g| sodium: 20mg

Cheesy Peach and Walnut Salad

Prep time: 10 minutes | Cook time: 0 minutes | Serves 1

1 ripe peach, pitted and sliced

¼ cup chopped walnuts, toasted

¼ cup shredded Parmesan cheese

1 teaspoon raw honey

Zest of 1 lemon

1 tablespoon chopped fresh mint

1. Combine the peach, walnut, and cheese in a medium bowl, then drizzle with honey. Spread the lemon zest and mint on top. Toss to combine everything well.
2. Serve immediately.

Per Serving

calories: 373 | fat: 26.4g | protein: 12.9g | carbs: 27.0g | fiber: 4.7g | sodium: 453mg

Greek Chicken, Tomato, and Olive Salad

Prep time: 10 minutes | Cook time: 0 minutes | Serves 2

Salad:

2 grilled boneless, skinless chicken breasts, sliced (about 1 cup)

10 cherry tomatoes, halved

8 pitted Kalamata olives, halved

½ cup thinly sliced red onion

Dressing:

¼ cup balsamic vinegar

1 teaspoon freshly squeezed lemon juice

¼ teaspoon sea salt

¼ teaspoon freshly ground black pepper

2 teaspoons extra-virgin olive oil

For Serving:

2 cups roughly chopped romaine lettuce

½ cup crumbled feta cheese

1. Combine the ingredients for the salad in a large bowl. Toss to combine well.
2. Combine the ingredients for the dressing in a small bowl. Stir to mix well.
3. Pour the dressing the bowl of salad, then toss to coat well. Wrap the bowl in plastic and refrigerate for at least 2 hours.

4. Remove the bowl from the refrigerator. Spread the lettuce on a large plate, then top with marinated salad. Scatter the salad with feta cheese and serve immediately.

Per Serving

calories: 328 | fat: 16.9g | protein: 27.6g | carbs: 15.9g | fiber: 3.1g| sodium: 1102mg

Ritzy Summer Fruit Salad

Prep time: 10 minutes | Cook time: 0 minutes | Serves 8

Salad:

1 cup fresh blueberries

2 cups cubed cantaloupe

2 cups red seedless grapes

1 cup sliced fresh strawberries

2 cups cubed honeydew melon

Zest of 1 large lime

½ cup unsweetened toasted coconut flakes

Dressing:

¼ cup raw honey

Juice of 1 large lime

¼ teaspoon sea salt

½ cup extra-virgin olive oil

1. Combine the ingredients for the salad in a large salad bowl, then toss to combine well.
2. Combine the ingredients for the dressing in a small bowl, then stir to mix well.
3. Dress the salad and serve immediately.

Per Serving

calories: 242 | fat: 15.5g | protein: 1.3g | carbs: 28.0g | fiber: 2.4g | sodium: 90mg

Sandwiches, Pizzas and Wraps

Falafel Balls with Tahini Sauce

Prep time: 2 hours 20 minutes | Cook time: 20 minutes | Serves 4

Tahini Sauce:

½ cup tahini

2 tablespoons lemon juice

¼ cup finely chopped flat-leaf parsley

2 cloves garlic, minced

½ cup cold water, as needed

Falafel:

1 cup dried chickpeas, soaked overnight, drained

¼ cup chopped flat-leaf parsley

¼ cup chopped cilantro

1 large onion, chopped

1 teaspoon cumin

½ teaspoon chili flakes

4 cloves garlic

1 teaspoon sea salt

5 tablespoons almond flour

1½ teaspoons baking soda, dissolved in 1 teaspoon water

2 cups peanut oil

1 medium bell pepper, chopped

1 medium tomato, chopped

4 whole-wheat pita breads

Make the Tahini Sauce

1. Combine the ingredients for the tahini sauce in a small bowl. Stir to mix well until smooth.
2. Wrap the bowl in plastic and refrigerate until ready to serve.

Make the Falafel

3. Put the chickpeas, parsley, cilantro, onion, cumin, chili flakes, garlic, and salt in a food processor. Pulse to mix well but not puréed.
4. Add the flour and baking soda to the food processor, then pulse to form a smooth and tight dough.
5. Put the dough in a large bowl and wrap in plastic. Refrigerate for at least 2 hours to let it rise.
6. Divide and shape the dough into walnut-sized small balls.
7. Pour the peanut oil in a large pot and heat over high heat until the temperature of the oil reaches 375ºF (190ºC).
8. Drop 6 balls into the oil each time, and fry for 5 minutes or until golden brown and crispy.

Turn the balls with a strainer to make them fried evenly.

9. Transfer the balls on paper towels with the strainer, then drain the oil from the balls.

10. Roast the pita breads in the oven for 5 minutes or until golden brown, if needed, then stuff the pitas with falafel balls and top with bell peppers and tomatoes. Drizzle with tahini sauce and serve immediately.

Per Serving

calories: 574 | fat: 27.1g | protein: 19.8g | carbs: 69.7g | fiber: 13.4g | sodium: 1246mg

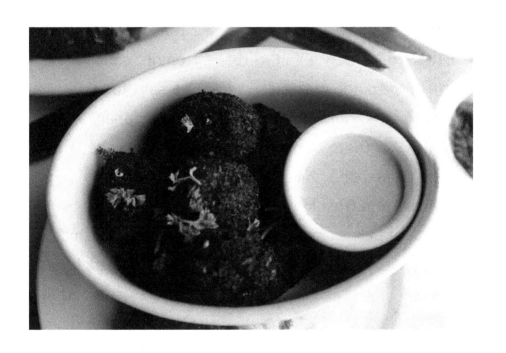

Glazed Mushroom and Vegetable Fajitas

Prep time: 20 minutes | Cook time: 20 minutes | Makes 6

Spicy Glazed Mushrooms:

1 teaspoon olive oil

1 (10- to 12-ounce / 284- to 340-g) package cremini mushrooms, rinsed and drained, cut into thin slices

½ to 1 teaspoon chili powder

Sea salt and freshly ground black pepper, to taste

1 teaspoon maple syrup

Fajitas:

2 teaspoons olive oil

1 onion, chopped

Sea salt, to taste

1 bell pepper, any color, deseeded and sliced into long strips

1 zucchini, cut into large matchsticks

6 whole-grain tortilla

2 carrots, grated

3 to 4 scallions, sliced

½ cup fresh cilantro, finely chopped

Make the Spicy Glazed Mushrooms

1. Heat the olive oil in a nonstick skillet over medium heat until shimmering.

2. Add the mushrooms and sauté for 10 minutes or until tender.

3. Sprinkle the mushrooms with chili powder, salt, and ground black pepper. Drizzle with maple syrup. Stir to mix well and cook for 5 to 7 minutes or until the mushrooms are glazed. Set aside until ready to use.

Make the Fajitas

4. Heat the olive oil in the same skillet over medium heat until shimmering.

5. Add the onion and sauté for 5 minutes or until translucent. Sprinkle with salt.

6. Add the bell pepper and zucchini and sauté for 7 minutes or until tender.

7. Meanwhile, toast the tortilla in the oven for 5 minutes or until golden brown.

8. Allow the tortilla to cool for a few minutes until they can be handled, then assemble the tortilla with glazed mushrooms, sautéed vegetables and remaining vegetables to make the fajitas. Serve immediately.

Per Serving

calories: 403 | fat: 14.8g | protein: 11.2g | carbs: 7.9g | fiber: 7.0g | sodium: 230mg

Cheesy Fig Pizzas with Garlic Oil

Prep time: 1 day 40 minutes | Cook time: 10 minutes | Makes 2 pizzas

Dough:

1 cup almond flour

1½ cups whole-wheat flour

¾ teaspoon instant or rapid-rise yeast

2 teaspoons raw honey

1¼ cups ice water

2 tablespoons extra-virgin olive oil

1¾ teaspoons sea salt

Garlic Oil:

4 tablespoons extra-virgin olive oil, divided

½ teaspoon dried thyme

2 garlic cloves, minced

⅛ teaspoon sea salt

½ teaspoon freshly ground pepper

Topping:

1 cup fresh basil leaves

1 cup crumbled feta cheese

8 ounces (227 g) fresh figs, stemmed and quartered lengthwise

2 tablespoons raw honey

Make the Dough

1. Combine the flours, yeast, and honey in a food processor, pulse to combine well. Gently add

water while pulsing. Let the dough sit for 10 minutes.

2. Mix the olive oil and salt in the dough and knead the dough until smooth. Wrap in plastic and refrigerate for at least 1 day.

Make the Garlic Oil

3. Heat 2 tablespoons of olive oil in a nonstick skillet over medium-low heat until shimmering.

4. Add the thyme, garlic, salt, and pepper and sauté for 30 seconds or until fragrant. Set them aside until ready to use.

Make the Pizzas

5. Preheat the oven to 500ºF (260ºC). Grease two baking sheets with 2 tablespoons of olive oil.

6. Divide the dough in half and shape into two balls. Press the balls into 13- inch rounds. Sprinkle the rounds with a tough of flour if they are sticky.

7. Top the rounds with the garlic oil and basil leaves, then arrange the rounds on the baking sheets. Scatter with feta cheese and figs.

8. Put the sheets in the preheated oven and bake for 9 minutes or until lightly browned. Rotate the pizza halfway through.

9. Remove the pizzas from the oven, then discard the bay leaves. Drizzle with honey. Let sit for 5 minutes and serve immediately.

Per Serving (1 pizza)

calories: 1350 | fat: 46.5g | protein: 27.5g | carbs: 221.9g | fiber: 23.7g | sodium: 2898mg

Mashed Grape Tomato Pizzas

Prep time: 10 minutes | Cook time: 20 minutes | Serves 6

3 cups grape tomatoes, halved

1 teaspoon chopped fresh thyme leaves

2 garlic cloves, minced

¼ teaspoon kosher salt

¼ teaspoon freshly ground black pepper

1 tablespoon extra-virgin olive oil

¾ cup shredded Parmesan cheese

6 whole-wheat pita breads

1. Preheat the oven to 425ºF (220ºC).
2. Combine the tomatoes, thyme, garlic, salt, ground black pepper, and olive oil in a baking pan.
3. Roast in the preheated oven for 20 minutes. Remove the pan from the oven, mash the tomatoes with a spatula and stir to mix well halfway through the cooking time.
4. Meanwhile, divide and spread the cheese over each pita bread, then place the bread in a separate baking pan and roast in the oven for

5 minutes or until golden brown and the cheese melts.

5. Transfer the pita bread onto a large plate, then top with the roasted mashed tomatoes. Serve immediately.

Per Serving

calories: 140 | fat: 5.1g | protein: 6.2g | carbs: 16.9g | fiber: 2.0g | sodium: 466mg

Vegetable and Cheese Lavash Pizza

Prep time: 15 minutes | Cook time: 11 minutes | Serves 4

2 (12 by 9-inch) lavash breads
2 tablespoons extra-virgin olive oil
10 ounces (284 g) frozen spinach, thawed and squeezed dry
1 cup shredded fontina cheese
1 tomato, cored and cut into ½-inch pieces
½ cup pitted large green olives, chopped
¼ teaspoon red pepper flakes
3 garlic cloves, minced
¼ teaspoon sea salt
¼ teaspoon ground black pepper
½ cup grated Parmesan cheese

1. Preheat oven to 475ºF (246ºC).
2. Brush the lavash breads with olive oil, then place them on two baking sheet. Heat in the preheated oven for 4 minutes or until lightly browned. Flip the breads halfway through the cooking time.

3. Meanwhile, combine the spinach, fontina cheese, tomato pieces, olives, red pepper flakes, garlic, salt, and black pepper in a large bowl. Stir to mix well.

4. Remove the lavash bread from the oven and sit them on two large plates, spread them with the spinach mixture, then scatter with the Parmesan cheese on top.

5. Bake in the oven for 7 minutes or until the cheese melts and well browned.

6. Slice and serve warm.

Per Serving

calories: 431 | fat: 21.5g | protein: 20.0g | carbs: 38.4g | fiber: 2.5g | sodium: 854mg

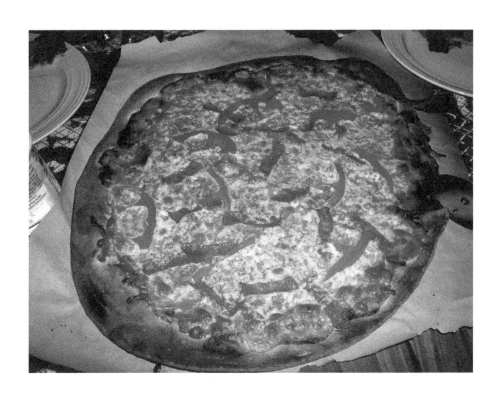

Dulse, Avocado, and Tomato Pitas

Prep time: 10 minutes | Cook time: 30 minutes | Makes 4 pitas

2 teaspoons coconut oil

½ cup dulse, picked through and separated

Ground black pepper, to taste

2 avocados, sliced

2 tablespoons lime juice

¼ cup chopped cilantro

2 scallions, white and light green parts, sliced

Sea salt, to taste

4 (8-inch) whole wheat pitas, sliced in half

4 cups chopped romaine

4 plum tomatoes, sliced

1. Heat the coconut oil in a nonstick skillet over medium heat until melted.

2. Add the dulse and sauté for 5 minutes or until crispy. Sprinkle with ground black pepper and turn off the heat. Set aside.

3. Put the avocado, lime juice, cilantro, and scallions in a food processor and sprinkle with salt and ground black pepper. Pulse to combine well until smooth.

4. Toast the pitas in a baking pan in the oven for 1 minute until soft.

5. Transfer the pitas to a clean work surface and open. Spread the avocado mixture over the pitas, then top with dulse, romaine, and tomato slices.

6. Serve immediately.

Per Serving (1 pita)

calories: 412 | fat: 18.7g | protein: 9.1g | carbs: 56.1g | fiber: 12.5g | sodium: 695mg

Greek Vegetable Salad Pita

Prep time: 10 minutes | Cook time: 0 minutes | Serves 4

½ cup baby spinach leaves

½ small red onion, thinly sliced

½ small cucumber, deseeded and chopped

1 tomato, chopped

1 cup chopped romaine lettuce

1 tablespoon extra-virgin olive oil

½ tablespoon red wine vinegar

1 teaspoon Dijon mustard

1 tablespoon crumbled feta cheese

Sea salt and freshly ground pepper, to taste

1 whole-wheat pita

1. Combine all the ingredients, except for the pita, in a large bowl. Toss to mix well.
2. Stuff the pita with the salad, then serve immediately.

Per Serving

calories: 137 | fat: 8.1g | protein: 3.1g | carbs: 14.3g | fiber: 2.4g | sodium: 166mg

Artichoke and Cucumber Hoagies

Prep time: 10 minutes | Cook time: 15 minutes | Makes 1

1 (12-ounce / 340-g) whole grain baguette, sliced in half horizontally

1 cup frozen and thawed artichoke hearts, roughly chopped

1 cucumber, sliced

2 tomatoes, sliced

1 red bell pepper, sliced

¼ cup Kalamata olives, pitted and chopped

¼ small red onion, thinly sliced

Sea salt and ground black pepper, to taste

2 tablespoons pesto

Balsamic vinegar, to taste

1. rrange the baguette halves on a clean work surface, then cut off the top third from each half. Scoop some insides of the bottom half out and reserve as breadcrumbs.
2. Toast the baguette in a baking pan in the oven for 1 minute to brown lightly.
3. Put the artichokes, cucumber, tomatoes, bell pepper, olives, and onion in a large bowl. Sprinkle with salt and ground black pepper. Toss to combine well.

4. Spread the bottom half of the baguette with the vegetable mixture and drizzle with balsamic vinegar, then smear the cut side of the baguette top with pesto. Assemble the two baguette halves.

5. Wrap the hoagies in parchment paper and let sit for at least an hour before serving.

Per Serving (1 hoagies)

calories: 1263 | fat: 37.7g | protein: 56.3g | carbs: 180.1g | fiber: 37.8g | sodium: 2137mg

Brown Rice and Black Bean Burgers

Prep time: 20 minutes | Cook time: 40 minutes | Makes 8 burgers

1 cup cooked brown rice

1 (15-ounce / 425-g) can black beans, drained and rinsed

1 tablespoon olive oil

2 tablespoons taco or Harissa seasoning

½ yellow onion, finely diced

1 beet, peeled and grated

1 carrot, peeled and grated

2 tablespoons no-salt-added tomato paste

2 tablespoons apple cider vinegar

3 garlic cloves, minced

¼ teaspoon sea salt

Ground black pepper, to taste

8 whole-wheat hamburger buns

Toppings:

16 lettuce leaves, rinsed well

8 tomato slices, rinsed well

Whole-grain mustard, to taste

1. Line a baking sheet with parchment paper.

2. Put the brown rice and black beans in a food processor and pulse until mix well. Pour the mixture in a large bowl and set aside.

3. Heat the olive oil in a nonstick skillet over medium heat until shimmering.

4. Add the taco seasoning and stir for 1 minute or until fragrant.

5. Add the onion, beet, and carrot and sauté for 5 minutes or until the onion is translucent and beet and carrot are tender.

6. Pour in the tomato paste and vinegar, then add the garlic and cook for 3 minutes or until the sauce is thickened. Sprinkle with salt and ground black pepper.

7. Transfer the vegetable mixture to the bowl of rice mixture, then stir to mix well until smooth.

8. Divide and shape the mixture into 8 patties, then arrange the patties on the baking sheet and refrigerate for at least 1 hour.

9. Preheat the oven to 400ºF (205ºC).

10. Remove the baking sheet from the refrigerator and allow to sit under room temperature for 10 minutes.

11. Bake in the preheated oven for 40 minutes or until golden brown on both sides. Flip the patties halfway through the cooking time.

12. Remove the patties from the oven and allow to cool for 10 minutes.

13. Assemble the buns with patties, lettuce, and tomato slices. Top the filling with mustard and serve immediately.

Per Serving (1 burger)

calories: 544 | fat: 20.0g | protein: 15.8g | carbs: 76.0g | fiber: 10.6g | sodium: 446mg

Classic Socca

Prep time: 10 minutes | Cook time: 10 minutes | Serves 4

1½ cups chickpea flour

½ teaspoon ground turmeric

½ teaspoon sea salt

½ teaspoon ground black pepper

2 tablespoons plus 2 teaspoons extra-virgin olive oil

1½ cups water

1. Combine the chickpea flour, turmeric, salt, and black pepper in a bowl. Stir to mix well, then gently mix in 2 tablespoons of olive oil and water. Stir to mix until smooth.
2. Heat 2 teaspoons of olive oil in an 8-inch nonstick skillet over medium- high heat until shimmering.
3. Add half cup of the mixture into the skillet and swirl the skillet so the mixture coat the bottom evenly.
4. Cook for 5 minutes or until lightly browned and crispy. Flip the socca halfway through the cooking time. Repeat with the remaining mixture.

5. Slice and serve warm.

Per Serving

calories: 207 | fat: 10.2g | protein: 7.9g | carbs: 20.7g | fiber: 3.9g | sodium: 315mg

Beans, Grains, and Pastas

Baked Rolled Oat with Pears and Pecans

Prep time: 15 minutes | Cook time: 30 minutes | Serves 6

2 tablespoons coconut oil, melted, plus more for greasing the pan

3 ripe pears, cored and diced

2 cups unsweetened almond milk

1 tablespoon pure vanilla extract

¼ cup pure maple syrup

2 cups gluten-free rolled oats

½ cup raisins

¾ cup chopped pecans

¼ teaspoon ground nutmeg

1 teaspoon ground cinnamon

½ teaspoon ground ginger

¼ teaspoon sea salt

1. Preheat the oven to 350ºF (180ºC). Grease a baking dish with melted coconut oil, then

spread the pears in a single layer on the baking dish evenly.

2. Combine the almond milk, vanilla extract, maple syrup, and coconut oil in a bowl. Stir to mix well.

3. Combine the remaining ingredients in a separate large bowl. Stir to mix well. Fold the almond milk mixture in the bowl, then pour the mixture over the pears.

4. Place the baking dish in the preheated oven and bake for 30 minutes or until lightly browned and set.

5. Serve immediately.

Per Serving

calories: 479 | fat: 34.9g | protein: 8.8g | carbs: 50.1g | fiber: 10.8g | sodium: 113mg

Brown Rice Pilaf with Pistachios and Raisins

Prep time: 5 minutes | Cook time: 15 minutes | Serves 6

1 tablespoon extra-virgin olive oil

1 cup chopped onion

½ cup shredded carrot

½ teaspoon ground cinnamon

1 teaspoon ground cumin

2 cups brown rice

1¾ cups pure orange juice

¼ cup water

½ cup shelled pistachios

1 cup golden raisins

½ cup chopped fresh chives

1. Heat the olive oil in a saucepan over medium-high heat until shimmering.
2. Add the onion and sauté for 5 minutes or until translucent.
3. Add the carrots, cinnamon, and cumin, then sauté for 1 minutes or until aromatic.
4. Pour int the brown rice, orange juice, and water. Bring to a boil. Reduce the heat to medium-low and simmer for 7 minutes or until the liquid is almost absorbed.

5. Transfer the rice mixture in a large serving bowl, then spread with pistachios, raisins, and chives. Serve immediately.

Per Serving

calories: 264 | fat: 7.1g | protein: 5.2g | carbs: 48.9g | fiber: 4.0g | sodium: 86mg

Cherry, Apricot, and Pecan Brown Rice Bowl

Prep time: 15 minutes | Cook time: 1 hour 1 minutes | Serves 2

2 tablespoons olive oil

2 green onions, sliced

½ cup brown rice

1 cup low -sodium chicken stock

2 tablespoons dried cherries

4 dried apricots, chopped

2 tablespoons pecans, toasted and chopped

Sea salt and freshly ground pepper, to taste

1. Heat the olive oil in a medium saucepan over medium-high heat until shimmering.
2. Add the green onions and sauté for 1 minutes or until fragrant.
3. Add the rice. Stir to mix well, then pour in the chicken stock.
4. Bring to a boil. Reduce the heat to low. Cover and simmer for 50 minutes or until the brown rice is soft.
5. Add the cherries, apricots, and pecans, and simmer for 10 more minutes or until the fruits are tender.

6. Pour them in a large serving bowl. Fluff with a fork. Sprinkle with sea salt and freshly ground pepper. Serve immediately.

Per Serving

calories: 451 | fat: 25.9g | protein: 8.2g | carbs: 50.4g | fiber: 4.6g | sodium: 122mg

Curry Apple Couscous with Leeks and Pecans

Prep time: 10 minutes | Cook time: 8 minutes | Serves 4

2 teaspoons extra-virgin olive oil

2 leeks, white parts only, sliced

1 apple, diced

2 cups cooked couscous

2 tablespoons curry powder

½ cup chopped pecans

1. Heat the olive oil in a skillet over medium heat until shimmering.
2. Add the leeks and sauté for 5 minutes or until soft.
3. Add the diced apple and cook for 3 more minutes until tender.
4. Add the couscous and curry powder. Stir to combine.
5. Transfer them in a large serving bowl, then mix in the pecans and serve.

Per Serving

calories: 254 | fat: 11.9g | protein: 5.4g | carbs: 34.3g | fiber: 5.9g | sodium: 15mg

Lebanese Flavor Broken Thin Noodles

Prep time: 10 minutes | Cook time: 25 minutes | Serves 6

1 tablespoon extra-virgin olive oil

1 (3-ounce / 85-g) cup vermicelli, broken into 1- to 1½-inch pieces

3 cups shredded cabbage

1 cup brown rice

3 cups low-sodium vegetable soup

½ cup water

2 garlic cloves, mashed

¼ teaspoon sea salt

⅛ teaspoon crushed red pepper flakes

½ cup coarsely chopped cilantro

Fresh lemon slices, for serving

1. Heat the olive oil in a saucepan over medium-high heat until shimmering.
2. Add the vermicelli and sauté for 3 minutes or until toasted.
3. Add the cabbage and sauté for 4 minutes or until tender.

4. Pour in the brown rice, vegetable soup, and water. Add the garlic and sprinkle with salt and red pepper flakes.
5. Bring to a boil over high heat. Reduce the heat to medium low. Put the lid on and simmer for another 10 minutes.
6. Turn off the heat, then let sit for 5 minutes without opening the lid.
7. Pour them on a large serving platter and spread with cilantro. Squeeze the lemon slices over and serve warm.

Per Serving

calories: 127 | fat: 3.1g | protein: 4.2g | carbs: 22.9g | fiber: 3.0g | sodium: 224mg

Lemony Farro and Avocado Bowl

Prep time: 5 minutes | Cook time: 25 minutes | Serves 4

1 tablespoon plus 2 teaspoons extra-virgin olive oil, divided

½ medium onion, chopped

1 carrot, shredded

2 garlic cloves, minced

1 (6-ounce / 170-g) cup pearled farro

2 cups low-sodium vegetable soup

2 avocados, peeled, pitted, and sliced

Zest and juice of 1 small lemon

¼ teaspoon sea salt

1. Heat 1 tablespoon of olive oil in a saucepan over medium-high heat until shimmering.
2. Add the onion and sauté for 5 minutes or until translucent.
3. Add the carrot and garlic and sauté for 1 minute or until fragrant.
4. Add the farro and pour in the vegetable soup. Bring to a boil over high heat. Reduce the heat to low. Put the lid on and simmer for 20 minutes or until the farro is al dente.
5. Transfer the farro in a large serving bowl, then fold in the avocado slices. Sprinkle with lemon

zest and salt, then drizzle with lemon juice and 2 teaspoons of olive oil.

6. Stir to mix well and serve immediately.

Per Serving

calories: 210 | fat: 11.1g | protein: 4.2g | carbs: 27.9g | fiber: 7.0g | sodium: 152mg

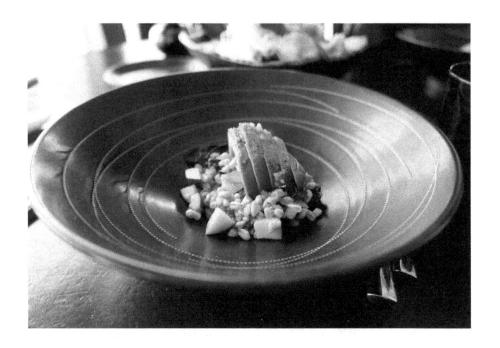

Rice and Blueberry Stuffed Sweet Potatoes

Prep time: 15 minutes | Cook time: 20 minutes | Serves 4

2 cups cooked wild rice

½ cup dried blueberries

½ cup chopped hazelnuts

½ cup shredded Swiss chard

1 teaspoon chopped fresh thyme

1 scallion, white and green parts, peeled and thinly sliced

Sea salt and freshly ground black pepper, to taste

4 sweet potatoes, baked in the skin until tender

1. Preheat the oven to 400ºF (205ºC).
2. Combine all the ingredients, except for the sweet potatoes, in a large bowl. Stir to mix well.
3. Cut the top third of the sweet potato off length wire, then scoop most of the sweet potato flesh out.
4. Fill the potato with the wild rice mixture, then set the sweet potato on a greased baking sheet.

5. Bake in the preheated oven for 20 minutes or until the sweet potato skin is lightly charred.

6. Serve immediately.

Per Serving

calories: 393 | fat: 7.1g | protein: 10.2g | carbs: 76.9g | fiber: 10.0g | sodium: 93mg

Slow Cooked Turkey and Brown Rice

Prep time: 20 minutes | Cook time: 3 hours 10 minutes | Serves 6

1 tablespoon extra-virgin olive oil

1½ pounds (680 g) ground turkey

2 tablespoons chopped fresh sage, divided

2 tablespoons chopped fresh thyme, divided

1 teaspoon sea salt

½ teaspoon ground black pepper

2 cups brown rice

1 (14-ounce / 397-g) can stewed tomatoes, with the juice

¼ cup pitted and sliced Kalamata olives

3 medium zucchini, sliced thinly

¼ cup chopped fresh flat-leaf parsley

1 medium yellow onion, chopped

1 tablespoon plus 1 teaspoon balsamic vinegar

2 cups low-sodium chicken stock

2 garlic cloves, minced

½ cup grated Parmesan cheese, for serving

1. Heat the olive oil in a nonstick skillet over medium-high heat until shimmering.

2. Add the ground turkey and sprinkle with 1 tablespoon of sage, 1 tablespoon of thyme, salt and ground black pepper.
3. Sauté for 10 minutes or until the ground turkey is lightly browned.
4. Pour them in the slow cooker, then pour in the remaining ingredients, except for the Parmesan. Stir to mix well.
5. Put the lid on and cook on high for 3 hours or until the rice and vegetables are tender.
6. Pour them in a large serving bowl, then spread with Parmesan cheese before serving.

Per Serving

calories: 499 | fat: 16.4g | protein: 32.4g | carbs: 56.5g | fiber: 4.7g | sodium: 758mg

Papaya, Jicama, and Peas Rice Bowl

Prep time: 20 minutes | Cook time: 45 minutes | Serves 4

Sauce:

Juice of ¼ lemon

2 teaspoons chopped fresh basil

1 tablespoon raw honey

1 tablespoon extra-virgin olive oil

Sea salt, to taste

Rice:

1½ cups wild rice

2 papayas, peeled, seeded, and diced

1 jicama, peeled and shredded

1 cup snow peas, julienned

2 cups shredded cabbage

1 scallion, white and green parts, chopped

1. Combine the ingredients for the sauce in a bowl. Stir to mix well. Set aside until ready to use.
2. Pour the wild rice in a saucepan, then pour in enough water to cover. Bring to a boil.
3. Reduce the heat to low, then simmer for 45 minutes or until the wild rice is soft and plump. Drain and transfer to a large serving bowl.

4. Top the rice with papayas, jicama, peas, cabbage, and scallion. Pour the sauce over and stir to mix well before serving.

Per Serving

calories: 446 | fat: 7.9g | protein: 13.1g | carbs: 85.8g | fiber: 16.0g | sodium: 70mg

Black Bean Chili with Mangoes

Prep time: 10 minutes | Cook time: 10 minutes | Serves 4

2 tablespoons coconut oil

1 onion, chopped

2 (15-ounce / 425-g) cans black beans, drained and rinsed

1 tablespoon chili powder

1 teaspoon sea salt

¼ teaspoon freshly ground black pepper

1 cup water

2 ripe mangoes, sliced thinly

¼ cup chopped fresh cilantro, divided

¼ cup sliced scallions, divided

1. Heat the coconut oil in a pot over high heat until melted.
2. Put the onion in the pot and sauté for 5 minutes or until translucent.
3. Add the black beans to the pot. Sprinkle with chili powder, salt, and ground black pepper. Pour in the water. Stir to mix well.
4. Bring to a boil. Reduce the heat to low, then simmering for 5 minutes or until the beans are tender.

5. Turn off the heat and mix in the mangoes, then garnish with scallions and cilantro before serving.

Per Serving

calories: 430 | fat: 9.1g | protein: 20.2g | carbs: 71.9g | fiber: 22.0g | sodium: 608mg

Poultry and Meats

Herbed-Mustard-Coated Pork Tenderloin

Prep time: 10 minutes | Cook time: 15 minutes | Serves 4

3 tablespoons fresh rosemary leaves

¼ cup Dijon mustard

½ cup fresh parsley leaves

6 garlic cloves

½ teaspoon sea salt

¼ teaspoon freshly ground black pepper

1 tablespoon extra-virgin olive oil

1 (1½-pound / 680-g) pork tenderloin

1. Preheat the oven to 400ºF (205ºC).
2. Put all the ingredients, except for the pork tenderloin, in a food processor. Pulse until it has a thick consistency.
3. Put the pork tenderloin on a baking sheet, then rub with the mixture to coat well.
4. Put the sheet in the preheated oven and bake for 15 minutes or until the internal temperature of the pork reaches at least 165ºF (74ºC). Flip

the tenderloin halfway through the cooking time.

5. Transfer the cooked pork tenderloin to a large plate and allow to cool for 5 minutes before serving.

Per Serving

calories: 363 | fat: 18.1g | protein: 2.2g | carbs: 4.9g | fiber: 2.0g | sodium: 514mg

Macadamia Pork

Prep time: 10 minutes | Cook time: 10 minutes | Serves 4

1 (1-pound / 454-g) pork tenderloin, cut into ½-inch slices and pounded thin

1 teaspoon sea salt, divided

¼ teaspoon freshly ground black pepper, divided

½ cup macadamia nuts

1 cup unsweetened coconut milk

1 tablespoon extra-virgin olive oil

1. Preheat the oven to 400ºF (205ºC).
2. On a clean work surface, rub the pork with ½ teaspoon of the salt and ⅛ teaspoon of the ground black pepper. Set aside.
3. Ground the macadamia nuts in a food processor, then combine with remaining salt and black pepper in a bowl. Stir to mix well and set aside.
4. Combine the coconut milk and olive oil in a separate bowl. Stir to mix well.

5. Dredge the pork chops into the bowl of coconut milk mixture, then dunk into the bowl of macadamia nut mixture to coat well. Shake the excess off.

6. Put the well-coated pork chops on a baking sheet, then bake for 10 minutes or until the internal temperature of the pork reaches at least 165ºF (74ºC).

7. Transfer the pork chops to a serving plate and serve immediately.

Per Serving

calories: 436 | fat: 32.8g | protein: 33.1g | carbs: 5.9g | fiber: 3.0g | sodium: 310mg

Grilled Chicken and Zucchini Kebabs

Prep time: 10 minutes | Cook time: 20 minutes | Serves 4

¼ cup extra-virgin olive oil

2 tablespoons balsamic vinegar

1 teaspoon dried oregano, crushed between your fingers

1 pound (454 g) boneless, skinless chicken breasts, cut into 1½-inch pieces

2 medium zucchinis, cut into 1-inch pieces

½ cup Kalamata olives, pitted and halved

2 tablespoons olive brine

¼ cup torn fresh basil leaves

Nonstick cooking spray

Special Equipment:

14 to 15 (12-inch) wooden skewers, soaked for at least 30 minutes

1. Spray the grill grates with nonstick cooking spray. Preheat the grill to medium-high heat.

2. In a small bowl, whisk together the olive oil, vinegar, and oregano. Divide the marinade between two large plastic zip-top bags.
3. Add the chicken to one bag and the zucchini to another. Seal and massage the marinade into both the chicken and zucchini.
4. Thread the chicken onto 6 wooden skewers. Thread the zucchini onto 8 or 9 wooden skewers.
5. Cook the kebabs in batches on the grill for 5 minutes, flip, and grill for 5 minutes more, or until any chicken juices run clear.
6. Remove the chicken and zucchini from the skewers to a large serving bowl. Toss with the olives, olive brine, and basil and serve.

Per Serving

calories: 283 | fat: 15.0g | protein: 11.0g | carbs: 26.0g | fiber: 3.0g | sodium: 575mg

Almond-Crusted Chicken Tenders with Honey

Prep time: 10 minutes | Cook time: 20 minutes | Serves 4

1 tablespoon honey

1 tablespoon whole-grain or Dijon mustard

¼ teaspoon freshly ground black pepper

¼ teaspoon kosher or sea salt

1 pound (454 g) boneless, skinless chicken breast tenders or tenderloins

1 cup almonds, roughly chopped

Nonstick cooking spray

1. Preheat the oven to 425ºF (220ºC). Line a large, rimmed baking sheet with parchment paper. Place a wire cooling rack on the parchment-lined baking sheet, and spray the rack well with nonstick cooking spray.

2. In a large bowl, combine the honey, mustard, pepper, and salt. Add the chicken and toss gently to coat. Set aside.

3. Dump the almonds onto a large sheet of parchment paper and spread them out. Press the coated chicken tenders into the nuts until

evenly coated on all sides. Place the chicken on the prepared wire rack.

4. Bake in the preheated oven for 15 to 20 minutes, or until the internal temperature of the chicken measures 165ºF (74ºC) on a meat thermometer and any juices run clear.

5. Cool for 5 minutes before serving.

Per Serving

calories: 222 | fat: 7.0g | protein: 11.0g | carbs: 29.0g | fiber: 2.0g | sodium: 448mg

Parsley-Dijon Chicken and Potatoes

Prep time: 5 minutes | Cook time: 22 minutes | Serves 6

1 tablespoon extra-virgin olive oil

1½ pounds (680 g) boneless, skinless chicken thighs, cut into 1-inch cubes, patted dry

1½ pounds (680 g) Yukon Gold potatoes, unpeeled, cut into ½-inch cubes

2 garlic cloves, minced

¼ cup dry white wine

1 cup low-sodium or no-salt-added chicken broth

1 tablespoon Dijon mustard

¼ teaspoon freshly ground black pepper

¼ teaspoon kosher or sea salt

1 cup chopped fresh flat-leaf (Italian) parsley, including stems

1 tablespoon freshly squeezed lemon juice

1. In a large skillet over medium-high heat, heat the oil. Add the chicken and cook for 5 minutes, stirring only after the chicken has browned on

one side. Remove the chicken and reserve on a plate.

2. Add the potatoes to the skillet and cook for 5 minutes, stirring only after the potatoes have become golden and crispy on one side. Push the potatoes to the side of the skillet, add the garlic, and cook, stirring constantly, for 1 minute. Add the wine and cook for 1 minute, until nearly evaporated. Add the chicken broth, mustard, salt, pepper, and reserved chicken. Turn the heat to high and bring to a boil.

3. Once boiling, cover, reduce the heat to medium-low, and cook for 10 to 12 minutes, until the potatoes are tender and the internal temperature of the chicken measures 165ºF (74ºC) on a meat thermometer and any juices run clear.

4. During the last minute of cooking, stir in the parsley. Remove from the heat, stir in the lemon juice, and serve.

Per Serving

calories: 324 | fat: 9.0g | protein: 16.0g | carbs: 45.0g | fiber: 5.0g | sodium: 560mg

Potato Lamb and Olive Stew

Prep time: 20 minutes | Cook time: 3 hours 42 minutes | Serves 10

4 tablespoons almond flour

¾ cup low-sodium chicken stock

1¼ pounds (567 g) small potatoes, halved

3 cloves garlic, minced

4 large shallots, cut into ½-inch wedges

3 sprigs fresh rosemary

1 tablespoon lemon zest

Coarse sea salt and black pepper, to taste

3½ pounds (1.6 kg) lamb shanks, fat trimmed and cut crosswise into 1½- inch pieces

2 tablespoons extra-virgin olive oil

½ cup dry white wine

1 cup pitted green olives, halved

2 tablespoons lemon juice

1. Combine 1 tablespoon of almond flour with chicken stock in a bowl. Stir to mix well.
2. Put the flour mixture, potatoes, garlic, shallots, rosemary, and lemon zest in the slow cooker.

Sprinkle with salt and black pepper. Stir to mix well. Set aside.

3. Combine the remaining almond flour with salt and black pepper in a large bowl, then dunk the lamb shanks in the flour and toss to coat.

4. Heat the olive oil in a nonstick skillet over medium-high heat until shimmering.

5. Add the well-coated lamb and cook for 10 minutes or until golden brown. Flip the lamb pieces halfway through the cooking time. Transfer the cooked lamb to the slow cooker.

6. Pour the wine in the same skillet, then cook for 2 minutes or until it reduces in half. Pour the wine in the slow cooker.

7. Put the slow cooker lid on and cook on high for 3 hours and 30 minutes or until the lamb is very tender.

8. In the last 20 minutes of the cooking, open the lid and fold in the olive halves to cook.

9. Pour the stew on a large plate, let them sit for 5 minutes, then skim any fat remains over the face of the liquid.

10. Drizzle with lemon juice and sprinkle with salt and pepper. Serve warm.

Per Serving

calories: 309 | fat: 10.3g | protein: 36.9g | carbs: 16.1g | fiber: 2.2g | sodium: 239mg

Slow Cook Lamb Shanks with Cannellini Beans Stew

Prep time: 20 minutes | Cook time: 10 hours 15 minutes | Serves 12

1 (19-ounce / 539-g) can cannellini beans, rinsed and drained

1 large yellow onion, chopped

2 medium-sized carrots, diced

1 large stalk celery, chopped

2 cloves garlic, thinly sliced

4 (1½-pound / 680-g) lamb shanks, fat trimmed

2 teaspoons tarragon

½ teaspoon sea salt

¼ teaspoon ground black pepper

1 (28-ounce / 794-g) can diced tomatoes, with the juice

1. Combine the beans, onion, carrots, celery, and garlic in the slow cooker. Stir to mix well.
2. Add the lamb shanks and sprinkle with tarragon, salt, and ground black pepper.
3. Pour in the tomatoes with juice, then cover the lid and cook on high for an hour.
4. Reduce the heat to low and cook for 9 hours or until the lamb is super tender.

5. Transfer the lamb on a plate, then pour the bean mixture in a colander over a separate bowl to reserve the liquid.

6. Let the liquid sit for 5 minutes until set, then skim the fat from the surface of the liquid. Pour the bean mixture back to the liquid.

7. Remove the bones from the lamb heat and discard the bones. Put the lamb meat and bean mixture back to the slow cooker. Cover and cook to reheat for 15 minutes or until heated through.

8. Pour them on a large serving plate and serve immediately.

Per Serving

calories: 317 | fat: 9.7g | protein: 52.1g | carbs: 7.0g | fiber: 2.1g | sodium: 375mg

Beef Kebabs with Onion and Pepper

Prep time: 15 minutes | Cook time: 10 minutes | Serves 6

2 pounds (907 g) beef fillet

1½ teaspoons salt

1 teaspoon freshly ground black pepper

½ teaspoon ground nutmeg

½ teaspoon ground allspice

⅛ cup extra-virgin olive oil

1 large onion, cut into 8 quarters

1 large red bell pepper, cut into 1-inch cubes

1. Preheat the grill to high heat.
2. Cut the beef into 1-inch cubes and put them in a large bowl.
3. In a small bowl, mix together the salt, black pepper, allspice, and nutmeg.
4. Pour the olive oil over the beef and toss to coat. Evenly sprinkle the seasoning over the beef and toss to coat all pieces.
5. Skewer the beef, alternating every 1 or 2 pieces with a piece of onion or bell pepper.

6. To cook, place the skewers on the preheated grill, and flip every 2 to 3 minutes until all sides have cooked to desired doneness, 6 minutes for medium-rare, 8 minutes for well done. Serve hot.

Per Serving

calories: 485 | fat: 36.0g | protein: 35.0g | carbs: 4.0g | fiber: 1.0g | sodium: 1453mg

Grilled Pork Chops

Prep time: 20 minutes | Cook time: 10 minutes | Serves 4

¼ cup extra-virgin olive oil

2 tablespoons fresh thyme leaves

1 teaspoon smoked paprika

1 teaspoon salt

4 pork loin chops, ½-inch-thick

1. In a small bowl, mix together the olive oil, thyme, paprika, and salt.
2. Put the pork chops in a plastic zip-top bag or a bowl and coat them with the spice mix. Let them marinate for 15 minutes.
3. Preheat the grill to high heat. Cook the pork chops for 4 minutes on each side until cooked through.
4. Serve warm.

Per Serving

calories: 282 | fat: 23.0g | protein: 21.0g | carbs: 1.0g | fiber: 0g | sodium: 832mg

Greek-Style Lamb Burgers

Prep time: 10 minutes | Cook time: 10 minutes | Serves 4

1 pound (454 g) ground lamb

½ teaspoon salt

½ teaspoon freshly ground black pepper

4 tablespoons crumbled feta cheese

Buns, toppings, and tzatziki, for serving (optional)

1. Preheat the grill to high heat.
2. In a large bowl, using your hands, combine the lamb with the salt and pepper.
3. Divide the meat into 4 portions. Divide each portion in half to make a top and a bottom. Flatten each half into a 3-inch circle. Make a dent in the center of one of the halves and place 1 tablespoon of the feta cheese in the center. Place the second half of the patty on top of the feta cheese and press down to close the 2 halves together, making it resemble a round burger.
4. Grill each side for 3 minutes, for medium-well. Serve on a bun with your favorite toppings and tzatziki sauce, if desired.

Per Serving

calories: 345 | fat: 29.0g | protein: 20.0g | carbs: 1.0g | fiber: 0g | sodium: 462mg

CPSIA information can be obtained
at www.ICGtesting.com
Printed in the USA
BVHW092216260621
610449BV00003B/700

9 781803 173955